This ***Tama Pasifika Wellbeing Journal*** is designed to help you to **CONNECT** back to yourself, strengthen your **TALANOA** skills and learn how to **HEAL** along your wellbeing journey.

"When we know who we are, own who we are and stand in our Pasifika potential - we are unstoppable."

Mani Malaeulu | co-author of Tama Sāmoa

CONNECT

**Connections are bonds that are formed
between people who feel seen,
heard and valued.
There are different kinds of connections
in our lives that help to let us know
that we matter.
But it is the self-connection,
our relationship with ourselves,
where we get to examine,
assess and reflect on our physical,
mental and spiritual needs.
In doing this, we are able to
better honour our needs and
form deeper connections with others,
our communities and the world.**

WHAT MAKES YOU, YOU?

Where were you born? Where have you lived?

What is your ethnicity
and what languages do you speak or want to speak?

Who do you live with? Who have you lived with?

What are you interested in?

What inspires you?

What is important to you and why?

What challenges have you faced?

What have you overcome?

MY STORY SO FAR ...

Think about what makes you, you, then use the space below to write or draw your life story so far:

Share your story
with someone.

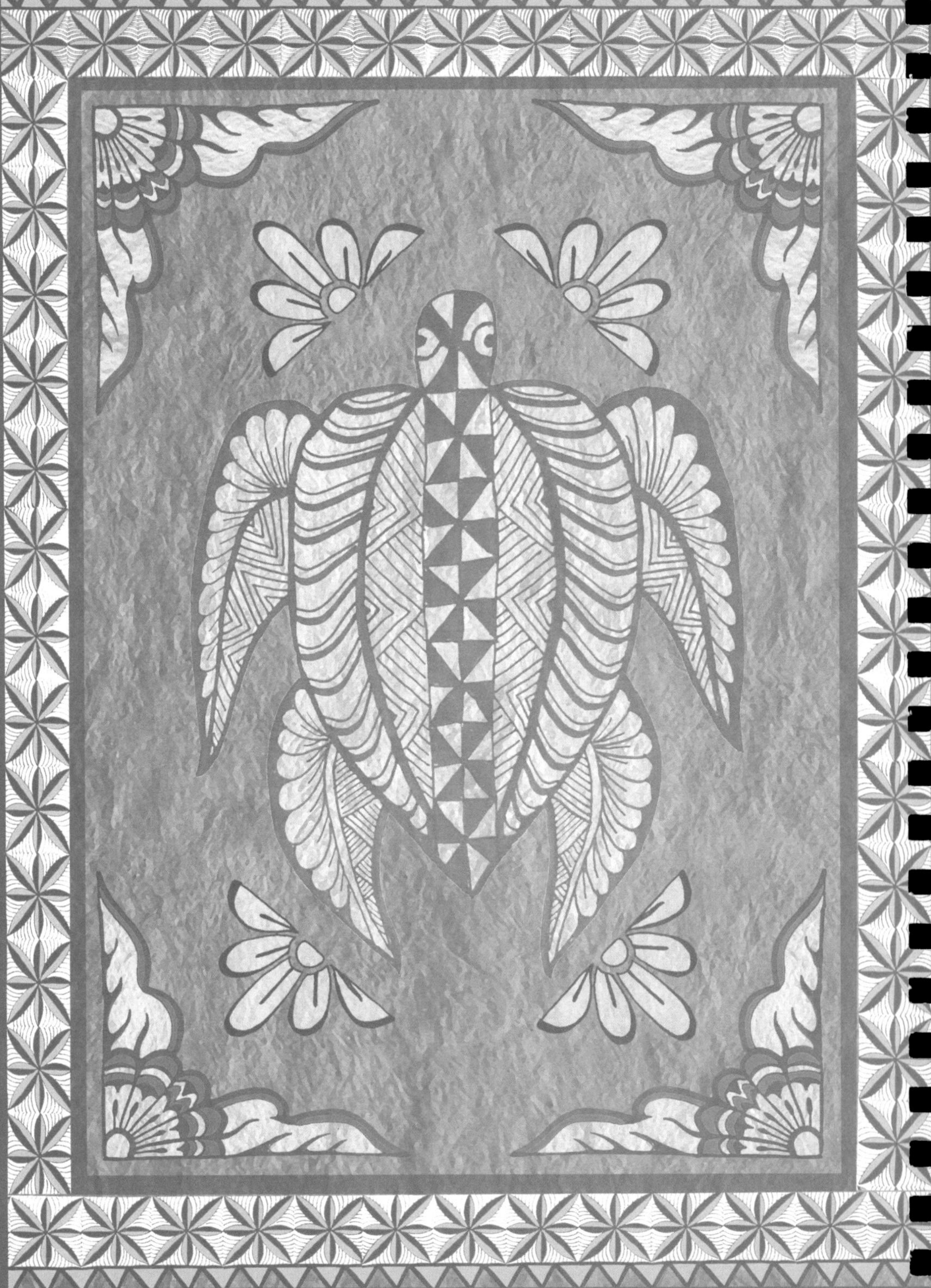

"And they wonder why we are so tight. We are connected through our Island bloodlines ... It's a connection between us that only we know. That makes us feel safe, understood and protected from the outside world ... I can be myself amongst my brothers and I don't have to be anyone or anything else. And I shouldn't have to be. None of us should. Facts."

Emmanuel Solomona | contributing author of Tama Sāmoa

OUR PASIFIKA STORY IN AOTEAROA SO FAR ...

Pacific health report calls for urgent system change amid massive inequities
SALE $4.00
Pacific languages fade in New Zealand
Polynesian athletes face stresses and strains in order to give back to families
Polynesian men a global sports commodity
Legacy: Celebrating 50 Years of Polynesian Panthers

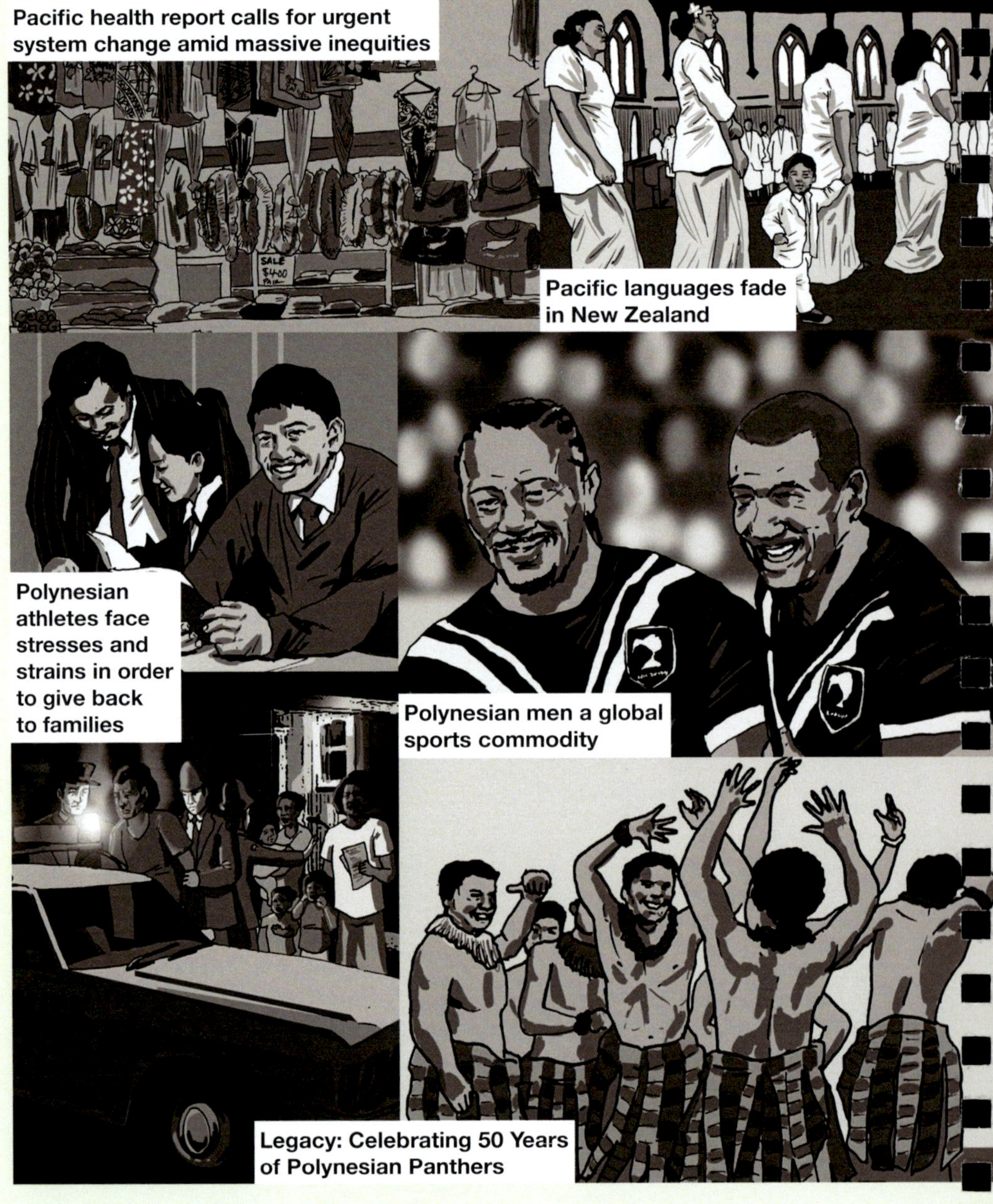

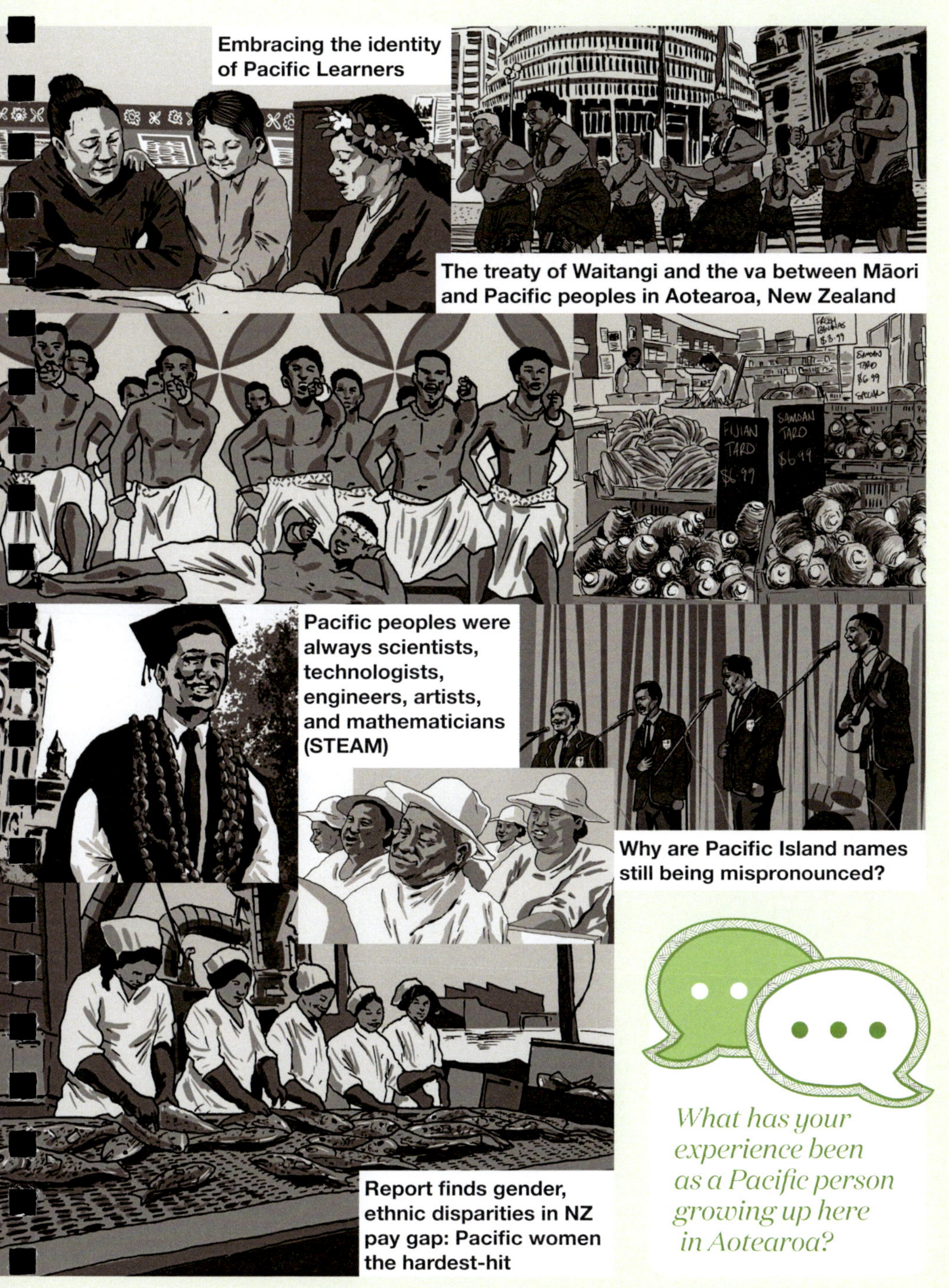
Embracing the identity of Pacific Learners
The treaty of Waitangi and the va between Māori and Pacific peoples in Aotearoa, New Zealand
FIJIAN TARO $6.99
SAMOAN TARO $6.99
Pacific peoples were always scientists, technologists, engineers, artists, and mathematicians (STEAM)
Why are Pacific Island names still being mispronounced?
Report finds gender, ethnic disparities in NZ pay gap: Pacific women the hardest-hit
What has your experience been as a Pacific person growing up here in Aotearoa?

TIME FOR A NEW STORY ...

What are your Pasifika Superpowers?

- ○ Acting in love
- ○ Pasifika proud
- ○ Being respectful
- ○ Humble
- ○ Serving and supporting others
- ○ Leading others
- ○ Never giving up, being resilient
- ○ Critical thinker, analyses and plans
- ○ Resourceful
- ○ Developing orator, knowing when and how to speak in different situations
- ○ Creative
- ○ Courageous and brave

Identify some areas you would like to work on:

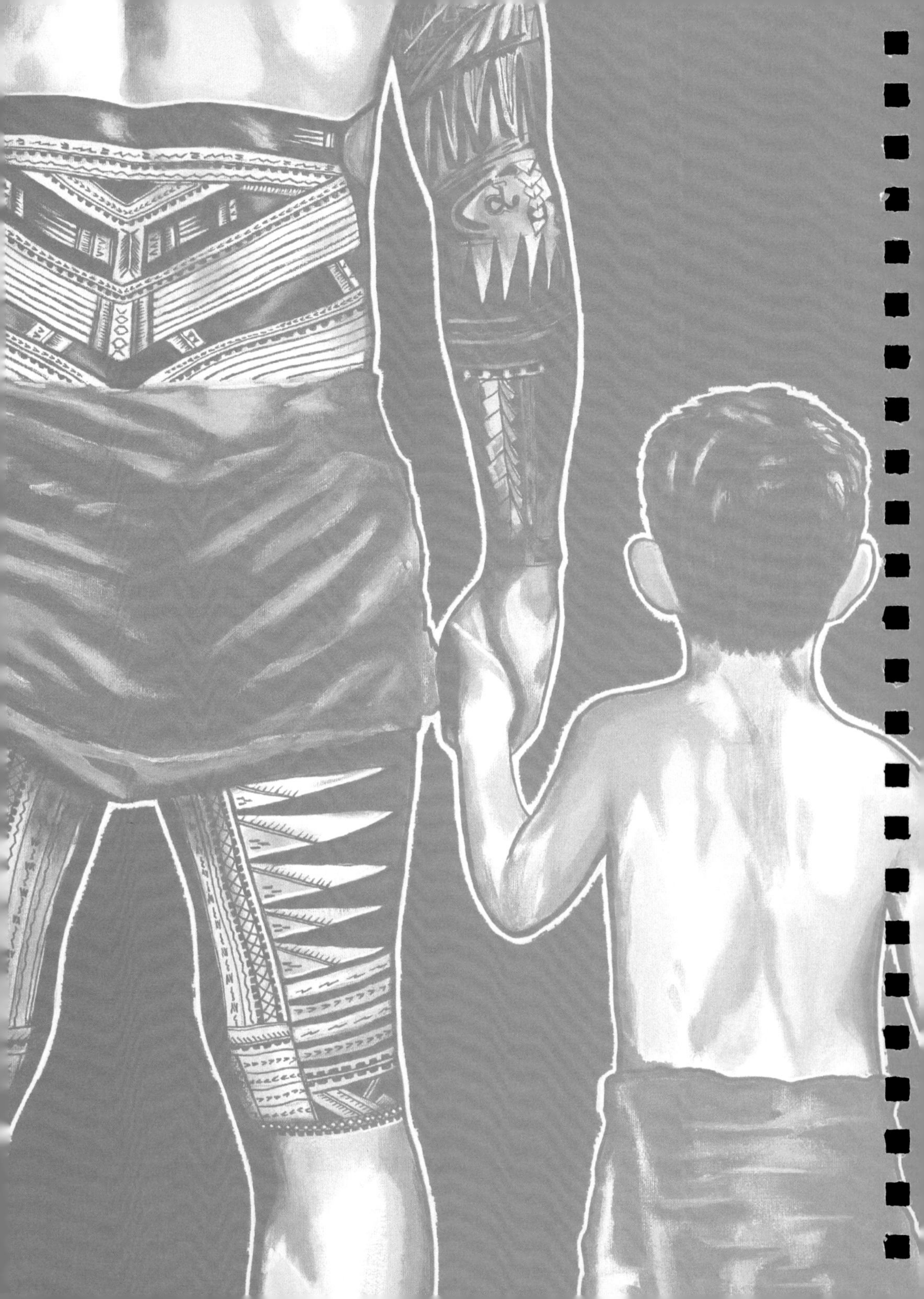

"Our ancestors guide and protect you
because a better life was their dream for us.
And that dream has not changed."

Atama Cassidy | contributing author of Tama Sāmoa

WHAT IS YOUR VISION FOR YOURSELF?

Draw your future self or something that represents your future and note down your dreams and goals.

TALANOA

**The power of talanoa,
conversation or communication
helps us to listen and hear
ourselves and others.
It is also the foundation of
connection and healing.
What we say and how we say things
helps us to explore our feelings
and express our needs.
This is why talanoa matters,
starting with the most important story
you will ever hear -
the story you tell yourself.**

POSITIVE TALK & NEGATIVE TALK

Self talk is the way you talk to yourself, or your inner voice. Everyone has one. Think about what you sometimes or always say to yourself and write it down here:

Our negative and positive thoughts can be powerful, but only if we give them power by believing and acting upon them. This is why learning to reframe our thoughts is important and has been proven to reduce stress, anxiety while helping us to develop resilience.

Reframing is simply changing the negative into a positive. Here's an example:

"I never get it right," can be reframed as
"I will learn from my mistakes and keep trying."

Try reframing any negative thoughts you have had using the grid below:

THOUGHT	NEGATIVE	REFRAMED THOUGHT

MANTRAS:

Mantras are phrases or statements we repeat to ourselves. They help to provide focus, mental clarity and enhance peace. Choose which mantras you could use or have used before:

- ○ I am worthy
- ○ I will be successful as who I am
- ○ I am enough
- ○ I am grateful
- ○ I can do this
- ○ I know what I am capable of
- ○ I am open to learning
- ○ I am creative and multi talented
- ○ I will grow from this
- ○ I am me
- ○ I can bounce back
- ○ I am needed
- ○ I deserve this
- ○ I accept myself and others as they are
- ○ I know who I am
- ○ I belong here

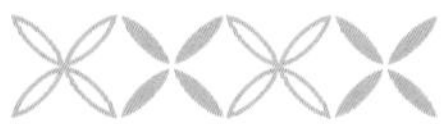

New mantras I can try ...

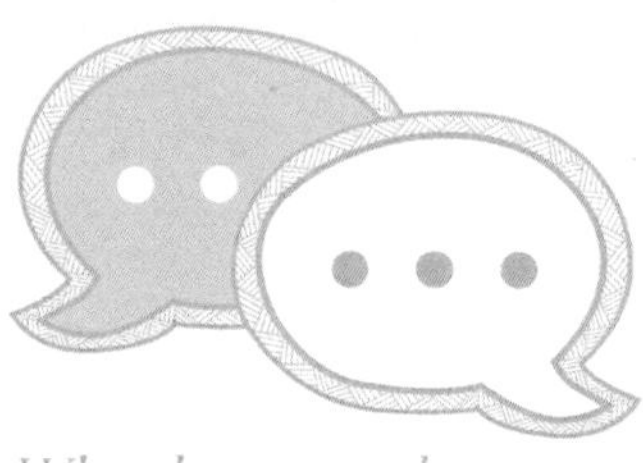

What have you learnt about self talk?

CONNECTING WITH OTHERS: RELATIONSHIPS

Connection gives us a sense of belonging while also giving purpose and meaning to our lives. Connection with others through positive relationships can lower anxiety and can improve self esteem and our immune system.

Think about the good relationships you have experienced and complete the sentence below:

I believe a good relationship includes these things ...

What relationships do I need to work on and why?

What can I do to improve these relationships?

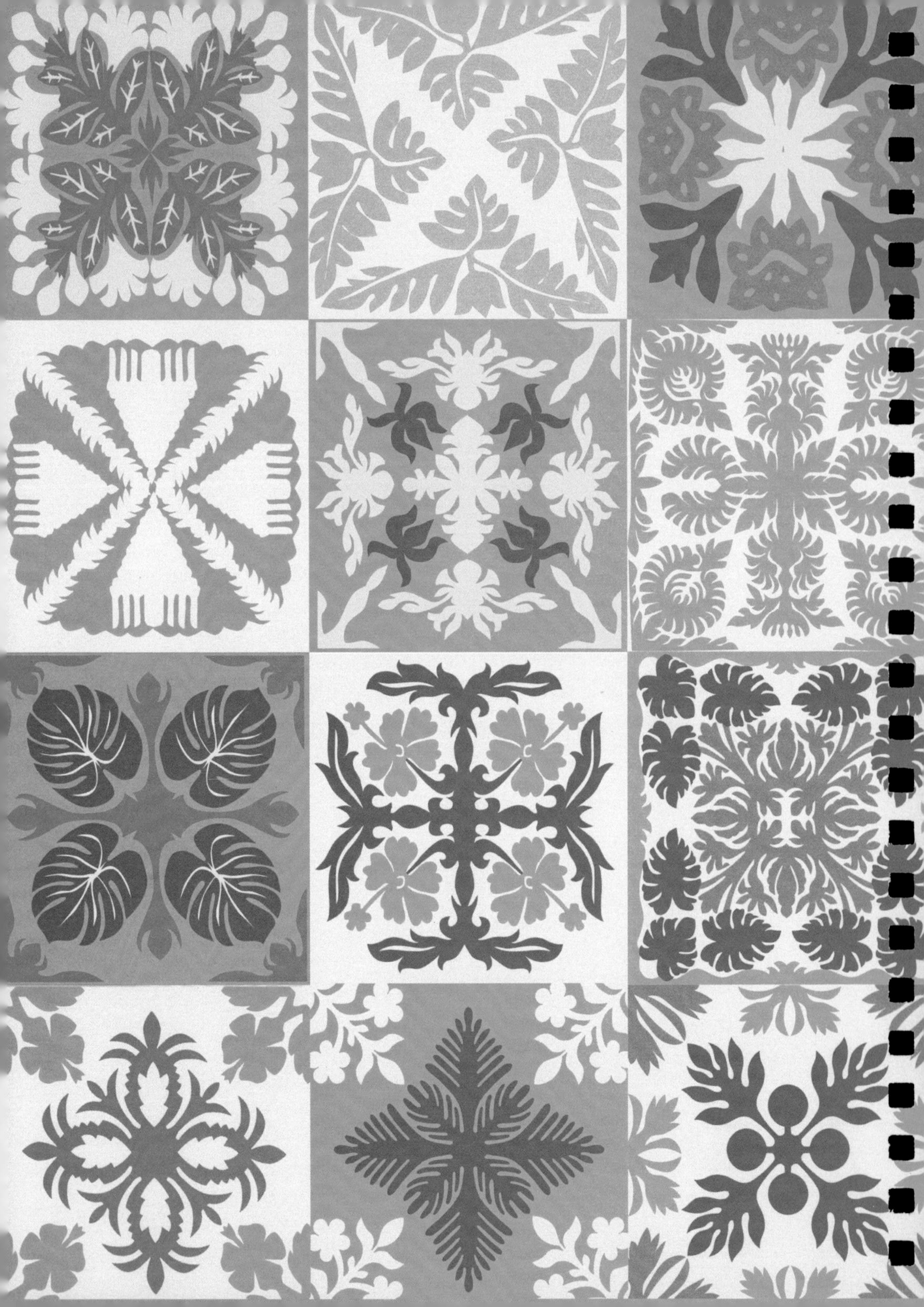

"By giving yourselves and each other permission to talk you have provided some amazing insights into your world that I hope will encourage you to have more talanoa."

Miss Duncan I Character from Tama Sāmoa

"Without realising it they had been working on opening up and reflecting on their lives, rediscovering and finding their voices. It was now time for them to be brave and to use it to reconnect with each other."

Tama Sāmoa quote

"... And now that you've found your voice, please never lose it."

Miss Va'a I Character from Tama Sāmoa

COURAGEOUS TALANOA

Challenges are a part of life with many situations requiring some courageous talanoa. A courageous talanoa involves the following elements:

Timing - Making sure everyone involved is ready to talk and is feeling safe.

Authentically honest - Sharing your experience by sticking to the facts and how the issue has impacted you.

Listen - Listening to understand not to react.

Accountablility - Accepting responsibility.

Next steps - Identifying what everyone will work on to make sure the issue does not happen again.

Opportunities - Confirming if there is a need for further support or future discussion.

Action apologies - Showing what sorry looks like through actions and following through on next steps.

Think about a courageous talanoa you have had and complete the following:

What was it about?

Was the issue resolved?

What helped?

What could you have done differently?

HEAL

Hurt and pain are a part of life which is why it is important to learn different ways to heal. Healing helps us to forgive, find peace and come back home to ourselves. It also makes us stronger and helps us to be more equipped to support others on their healing journeys.

SELF CARE

Self care can be difficult sometimes since it can be viewed as being self serving instead or serving others which is a major part of our Pasifika cultures. But self care is essential in helping us to be the best versions of ourselves, which in turn helps us to be better for others. Complete the activity below:

What do you do to take care of yourself?

PHYSICAL	MENTAL	SPIRITUAL
○ Exercise	○ Read	○ Pray
○ Sports	○ Stay connected with others	○ Go to Church
○ Walk/Move	○ Relax	○ Sing
○ Dance	○ Alone time	○ Dance
○ Sing	○ Time in Nature	○ Writing
○ Creative Activity	○ Set goals	○ Meditation
○ Stay Hydrated	○ Visualization	○ Time in Nature
○ Eat healthy foods		○ Quiet time

OTHER:

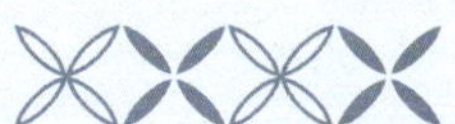

Here are some things I want to work on to take better care of myself ...

GRATITUDE

Being thankful each day for the good things in our lives helps us to always look at the bright side of things. Other reasons include:

Helps us to be present.

More positive and optimistic.

Deal with challenges better.

More resilient.

Lifts mood.

Boosts energy.

Decreases stress and anxiety.

Improves self esteem.

What are the top 3 things you are grateful for right now:

1. I am grateful for ...

   because ...

2. I am grateful for ...

   because ...

3. I am grateful for ...

   because ...

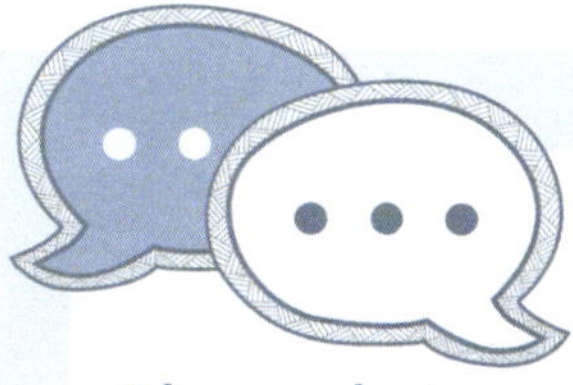

Share what you are grateful for with another person.

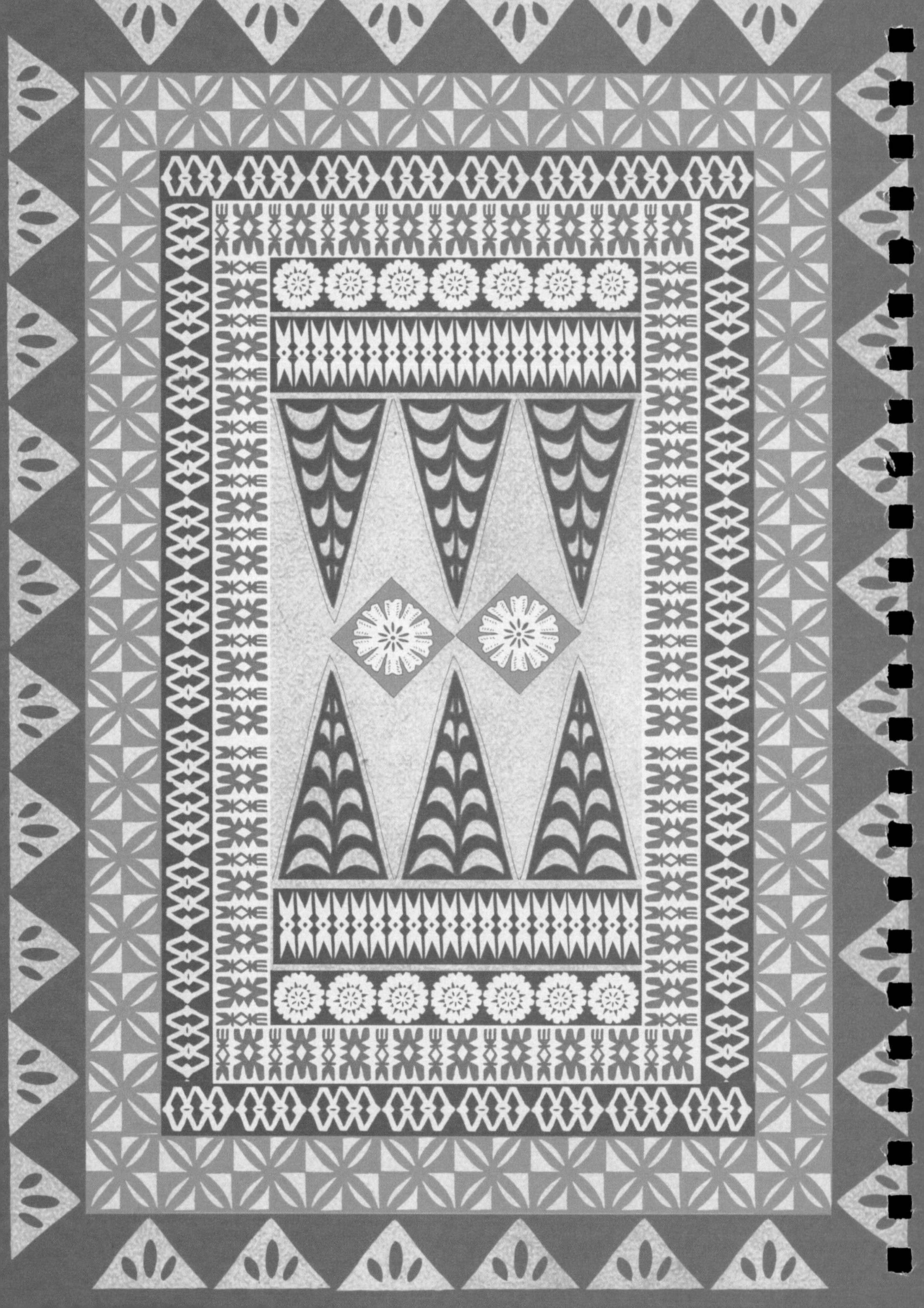

*“if you choose the ‘harden up’
and hold it in option,
I reckon it usually comes
out another way.”*

Aleki Leala | Contributing author of Tama Sāmoa

LETTING GO

Acceptance, forgiveness, controlling what we can control helps us to heal and let go of what might be holding us back.
Letting go means setting yourself free.

What do you need to let go of?

- A bad relationship
- Not receiving that apology you feel you deserve
- Losing a loved one
- Trauma
- An experience of failure
- Guilt
- Being treated differently
- Shame
- Being disrespected
- Fear of being who you really are
- Not valued
- Judgement
- Someone making a false assumption of you
- Violence or abuse

Here are some tips for letting go:

Acknowledge what happened, happened.

Take ownership in your part of the hurt that took place.

Channel your focus on something positive.

Control what you can control.

Allow yourself to feel.

Find something you can be grateful for.

Pray. Pray. Pray. Pray.

Start exercise practice.

Surround yourself with people that love you, will be honest with you and encourage you.

Eat healthy foods.

Be kind to yourself.

Forgive yourself, you're only human.

Breathing and taking time for yourself.

MY TEAM

It is important to surround ourselves with people who are there for us in the fun times AND the hard times.

Who are these people in your life?

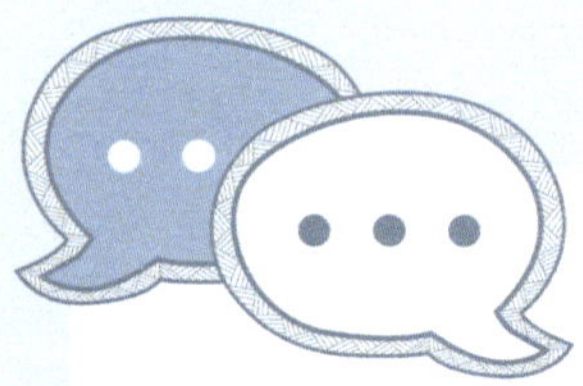

We become the people we surround ourselves with. Think about this statement and share your thoughts with someone.

Below is a list of some of the services available in Aotearoa that offer support, information and help for you, your parents, family and friends.

1737 - Need to talk?
Free call or text 1737 anytime, to talk to a trained counsellor.

Youthline
Call 0800 376 633 or free text 234 for 12-24 year olds.

What's Up
Call 0800 942 8787 or use the online chat at www.whatsup.co.nz for 5-18 year olds.

For more useful information and support visit **www.LeVa.co.nz**

HEALING FOR ME ...

Sounds like

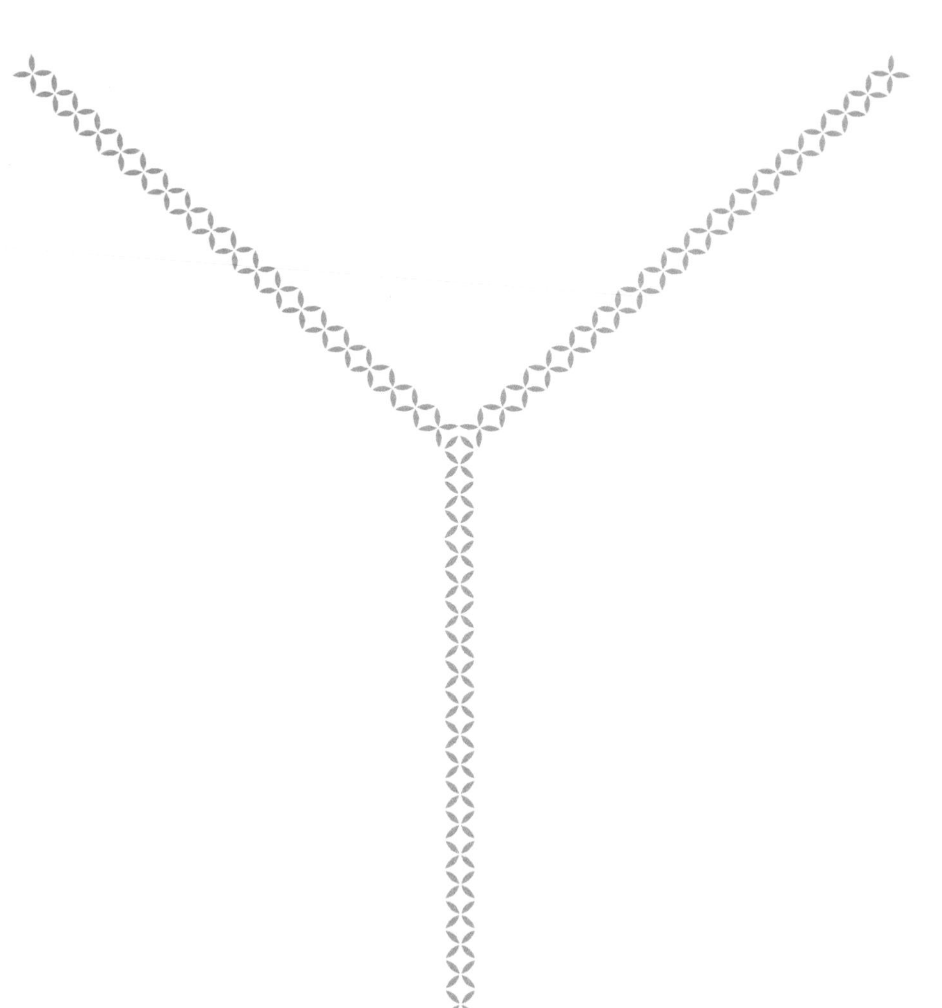

Looks like

Feels like

... the lessons for us are always in the journey not the destination."

Mikaele Savali | Contributing author of Tama Sāmoa

DEAR USO...

Write a letter to your younger self. What are the things you would say to help encourage, uplift and heal from the experiences that you will go through?

Dear Uso,

NEXT STEPS:

Look back in your wellbeing journal
and note your goals down for each section:

CONNECT ... Vision for yourself?

TALANOA ... Talanoa goals?

HEAL ... Healing strategies?

What action steps will you take to help you achieve these goals?

STEPS TO CONNECT

STEPS TO TALANOA

STEPS TO HEAL

Complete the following journal entries to help you monitor your progress and assess your needs along your wellbeing journey.

WEEK 1

What are the highlights? Your wins this week? Feelings? Any challenges? Help or support needed? New learnings?

CONNECT

TALANOA

HEAL

Noticings, Wonderings, Thoughts, Ideas, Breakthroughs ...

"When others see us, I want them to see so many possibilities and potential. I want them to know that our parents have worked so hard and sacrificed so much for us to be more than the stereotypes we face growing up."

Senio Sanele | Contributing author of Tama Sāmoa

WEEK 2

What are the highlights? Your wins this week? Feelings? Any challenges? Help or support needed? New learnings?

CONNECT

TALANOA

HEAL

Noticings, Wonderings, Thoughts, Ideas, Breakthroughs ...

---

*"So keep rising like the stars our ancestors used to sail
the great Pacific Ocean, be the master of your journey
to take control of our destination, for you, and for all of us ..."*

Emmanuel Solomona | Contributing author of Tama Sāmoa

WEEK 3

What are the highlights? Your wins this week? Feelings? Any challenges? Help or support needed? New learnings?

CONNECT

TALANOA

HEAL

Noticings, Wonderings, Thoughts, Ideas, Breakthroughs ...

"It can be so hard for us boys sometimes, because it's just how it's always been I guess - not talking, bottling it all up, this idea of being a man. But just because it's always been this way it doesn't mean it's right."

Aleki Leala | Contributing author of Tama Sāmoa

WEEK 4

What are the highlights? Your wins this week? Feelings? Any challenges? Help or support needed? New learnings?

CONNECT

TALANOA

HEAL

Noticings, Wonderings, Thoughts, Ideas, Breakthroughs ...

---

*"But as I succeeded and found who I was;
I knew you both saw it too. When you realised that
all you wanted was for me to be happy
– that was the day I knew I was good enough."*

Okirano Fialele | Contributing author of Tama Sāmoa

WEEK 5

What are the highlights? Your wins this week? Feelings? Any challenges? Help or support needed? New learnings?

CONNECT

TALANOA

HEAL

Noticings, Wonderings, Thoughts, Ideas, Breakthroughs ...

"To whoever reads my story, I hope this brings light to the darkness you may be going through. I hope it gives clarity in the chaos that we all must face at times in our life. And I hope you understand that the pain you may be going through right now, cannot compare to the joy that is coming."

Israel Risati Sua-Taulelei | Contributing author of Tama Sāmoa

WEEK 6

What are the highlights? Your wins this week? Feelings? Any challenges? Help or support needed? New learnings?

CONNECT

TALANOA

HEAL

Noticings, Wonderings, Thoughts, Ideas, Breakthroughs ...

"I can be quiet. Sometimes too quiet.
But I have thoughts, feelings, and ideas too."

Isaac Sanele | Contributing author of Tama Sāmoa

WEEK 7

What are the highlights? Your wins this week? Feelings? Any challenges? Help or support needed? New learnings?

CONNECT

TALANOA

HEAL

Noticings, Wonderings, Thoughts, Ideas, Breakthroughs ...

"Success is a package deal for our Tama Pasifika.
To connect with us is to connect with our families.
To connect with our families leads to connecting with our culture."

Liko Alosio | Contributing author of Tama Sāmoa

WEEK 8

What are the highlights? Your wins this week? Feelings? Any challenges? Help or support needed? New learnings?

CONNECT

TALANOA

HEAL

Noticings, Wonderings, Thoughts, Ideas, Breakthroughs ...

"... there is real value in viewing the world through a duel lens, and when guided with fa'aaloalo (respect), fa'amaoni (honesty), usita'i (discipline), plus the potential we possess as Pasifika, we really are unstoppable."

Mikaele Savali | Contributing author of Tama Sāmoa

WEEK 9

What are the highlights? Your wins this week? Feelings? Any challenges? Help or support needed? New learnings?

CONNECT

TALANOA

HEAL

Noticings, Wonderings, Thoughts, Ideas, Breakthroughs ...

"Change takes time and this is why you are needed for the change to happen ... Your difference is what will make the difference."

Atama Cassidy | Contributing author of Tama Sāmoa

WEEK 10

What are the highlights? Your wins this week? Feelings? Any challenges? Help or support needed? New learnings?

CONNECT

TALANOA

HEAL

Noticings, Wonderings, Thoughts, Ideas, Breakthroughs ...

---

*"No more, See-through. For me.
My language. Anchors me ... When help arrives. I know.
Tides will turn. Full. Solid. I'll be complete."*

Elijah Solomona | Contributing author of Tama Sāmoa

WEEK 11

What are the highlights? Your wins this week? Feelings? Any challenges? Help or support needed? New learnings?

CONNECT

TALANOA

HEAL

Noticings, Wonderings, Thoughts, Ideas, Breakthroughs ...

"I realize that going forward, this is my journey, that I am now fully committed to and own ..."

Saul Luamanuvae-Su'a | Contributing author of Tama Sāmoa

WEEK 12

What are the highlights? Your wins this week? Feelings? Any challenges? Help or support needed? New learnings?

CONNECT

TALANOA

HEAL

Noticings, Wonderings, Thoughts, Ideas, Breakthroughs ...

"Hold fast to the cultural values and lessons you have been taught. These must never change. It is the world around you that will. Prepare for the tides to change and know that our original wayfinders, your ancestors, are with you all the way."

Atama Cassidy | Contributing author of Tama Sāmoa

DEAR USO,

Write a letter to the future you, what would you say to him knowing what you now know. *What would be some of things that you would be most proud of? What is he like and how has he inspired you? Who has this young man become? How has he honoured himself, his family and other people in his life?*

Notes:

Notes:

Notes:

Notes:

"When you succeed as Pasifika we all succeed as Pasifika."

Mani Malaeulu | Co-author of Tama Sāmoa